YUP, YOUR UTERUS CAN FALL OUT AS YOU GET OLDER

A Holistic Approach to Uterine Prolapse Insights

Ruth M. Smith

Table of Contents

Chapter 1

<u>UNDERSTANDING UTERINE PROLAPSE</u>

Uterine prolapse is a disease where the muscles and tissues around your uterus become weak. This causes your uterus to sag or drop down into your vagina. It can happen to anyone assigned female at birth (AFAB) but is most frequent after menopause and in folks who've had more than one vaginal delivery.

The uterus (womb) is an organ of the female reproductive system. It is fashioned like an upside-down pear and is positioned inside the pelvis.

The uterus, bladder, and colon are supported by a hammock of muscles situated between the tailbone (coccyx) and the pubic bone within the pelvis. These muscles are known as the pelvic floor, or the levator ani muscles.

Uterine prolapse is a frequent ailment that might arise as a person matures. Over time, and with multiple vaginal childbirths, the muscles and ligaments around your uterus weaken. When this support structure starts to weaken, your uterus can sag out of position.

The muscles, ligaments, and tissues in your pelvis are called your pelvic floor muscles. These muscles support your uterus, rectum, vagina, bladder, and other pelvic organs.

A prolapse occurs when your pelvic floor muscles are injured or weakened to the point where they can no longer supply support. This causes your pelvic organs to drop into or out of your vagina.

Uterine prolapse can be modest or severe depending on how weak the supporting muscles of your uterus have become. In an incomplete prolapse, your uterus may have slipped sufficiently to be partway into your vagina.

This generates a hump or bulge. In a more severe case, your uterus can slip far enough that it comes out of your vagina. This is called a complete prolapse.

What are the phases of uterine prolapse?

Your healthcare practitioner may use a system to classify uterine prolapse. The phases of uterine prolapse are:

Stage 0: No Prolapse (Asymptomatic)

In this stage, there is no prolapse or sinking of the uterus into the vaginal canal. Women may not suffer any symptoms, and the uterus continues in its regular anatomical position.

Stage I: Mild Prolapse (Cystocele)

In this stage, the uterus is slightly descended into the upper region of the vaginal canal. The cervix is still within the vaginal canal, and the uterus may be touched with a pelvic exam. Some women could feel symptoms like a sensation of pressure or fullness in the pelvic area, particularly after standing for extended durations.

Stage II: Moderate Prolapse (Cystocele and Rectocele)

In this stage, the descent of the uterus is more obvious. The cervix may extend into or slightly beyond the vaginal opening. Along with uterine descent, there may also be related cystoceles (bladder prolapse) and rectocele (rectal prolapse).

Troubles may include vaginal pressure, a feeling of something coming out of the vagina, discomfort during intercourse, and urine or bowel troubles.

Stage III: Severe Prolapse (Procidentia)

At this stage, the uterus is substantially depressed and may protrude outside the vaginal entrance, which is also known as procidentia. This stage frequently contains a combination of uterine, bladder, and rectal prolapse.

Women may experience more pronounced symptoms such as urine incontinence, difficulty emptying the bladder or bowels, and discomfort or pain.

Stage IV: Complete Prolapse (Procidentia)

In this advanced stage, the uterus, bladder, and rectum have descended to the point where they protrude outside the vaginal opening. The uterus may appear like a bulging lump.

Women with full prolapse may encounter severe discomfort and functional difficulties, including trouble with urine, bowel movements, and sexual intercourse.

Who gets uterine prolapse?

Uterine prolapse is most likely to happen in those who:

- Have had one or more vaginal deliveries.
- Have reached menopause.
- Have a family history of uterine prolapse.
- Have undergone prior pelvic surgeries.

Menopause comes when your ovaries cease generating the hormones that govern your monthly menstrual flow. One of these hormones is oestrogen. This particular hormone helps keep your pelvic muscles strong. Without it, you're at a higher risk of suffering a prolapse.

How prevalent is uterine prolapse?
Uterine prolapse is a very frequent condition. Your risk of developing the ailment increases with age. You're also at a larger risk of uterine prolapses if you've had many vaginal deliveries.

How serious is a prolapsed uterus?
Uterine prolapse can hamper daily activities and be uncomfortable. Very mild cases may not require treatment or cause any discomfort. However, severe cases may make it difficult to pee or have a proper bowel movement.

Uterine prolapse is often a quality-of-life concern, and healthcare providers address it when symptoms of the disorder begin to interfere with your normal life.

What conditions are related to uterine prolapse?

Other organs in your pelvic region can fall out of position when the muscles around it become too weak. Some of the other types of pelvic organ prolapse are:

<u>Cystocele</u>: When your bladder drops into or out of your vagina.

<u>Rectocele:</u> When your rectum bulges into or out of your vagina.

<u>Enterocele:</u> When a part of your small intestine bulges into your vagina.

What happens if a prolapsed uterus is left untreated?

It depends on the severity of the prolapse. In small circumstances where your quality of life isn't harmed, your healthcare practitioner may not propose therapy.

Uterine prolapse can affect other organs in the pelvic area of your body (such as your bladder and rectum). Healthcare providers generally urge treatment when uterine prolapse becomes unpleasant.

Can I push my prolapsed uterus back up?

No, you can't push your uterus back up. Only your healthcare provider can treat a prolapsed uterus.

Can uterine prolapse happen again?

Most of the time, treatment for uterine prolapse is beneficial. But sometimes, a prolapse could come back. This is more common if you:

- Have a really serious prolapse.
- Have obesity.
- Are younger than 60.

What's the outlook for uterine prolapse?

In most circumstances, the outlook for uterine prolapse is very bright. Seeking treatment and following lifestyle improvements (maintaining a healthy weight and exercising) can help prevent a prolapse from developing again.

Talk to your healthcare practitioner about any concerns you may have concerning prolapses. Your practitioner can assist build a treatment plan and support good lifestyle practices to prevent any future prolapses.

Can one get pregnant with uterine prolapse?

But women of child-bearing age can also have a prolapse, which poses the question surrounding becoming pregnant with uterine prolapse. The short answer is yes, pregnancy during uterine prolapse is achievable.

Does the prolapsed uterus go back to normal?

In some ladies, it can become better with time. It's crucial to look at causes, symptoms, therapies, and everyday things you may perform to prevent/improve prolapse.

Can you have another baby after a prolapse?

If you still have vaginal prolapse when you subsequently get pregnant, you may require particular care from your medical team. Pregnancy and birth are not the only variables that affect your pelvic floor. Your own circumstances can cause complications, including: being constipated: straining is not healthy for your pelvic floor.

Can a prolapsed uterus cause miscarriage?

Uterine prolapse during pregnancy is a rare disorder. It can cause premature labour, spontaneous abortion, foetal demise, maternal urinary issue, maternal sepsis, and mortality.

Can you feel a uterine prolapse with your finger?

How can I feel a prolapsed uterus with my finger? Insert 1 or 2 fingers and position them over the front vaginal wall (facing the bladder) to feel any bulging under your fingertips, initially with violent coughing and then with prolonged bearing down.

<u>CAUSES</u>

Your uterus is held in place within your pelvis by a combination of muscles and ligaments (pelvic floor muscles). When these structures weaken, they become unable to hold your uterus in position and it begins to sag. Several factors can contribute to the weakening of the pelvic muscles, including:

1. **Weak Pelvic Floor Muscles:** One of the key reasons for uterine prolapse is weaker pelvic floor muscles. These muscles provide a critical purpose in maintaining the uterus, bladder, and rectum.

Factors that can lead to muscle weakness include ageing, pregnancy, hormonal changes (such as a fall in oestrogen levels after menopause), and chronic straining from conditions like constipation or heavy lifting.

2. **Childbirth and Trauma:** The act of giving birth can place considerable stress on the pelvic floor muscles and ligaments. Multiple childbirths, especially if the deliveries were traumatic or featured large babies, can increase the incidence of uterine prolapse.

Vaginal birth, particularly if it's protracted or involves forceps or vacuum extraction, can lead to straining and weakening of the pelvic tissues.

3. **Hormonal Changes:** Oestrogen is a hormone that helps maintain the health and flexibility of pelvic tissues, notably the muscles, and ligaments supporting the uterus.

A decline in oestrogen levels, as seen after menopause, can contribute to the weakening of these tissues and elevate the risk of prolapse.

4. **Genetic Predisposition:** Some study reveals that there might be a genetic susceptibility to pelvic floor weakness and uterine prolapse. If other women in your family have experienced prolapse, you may be at a higher risk.

5. Chronic Straining and Pressure:
Chronic straining during bowel motions owing to constipation can impose undue pressure on the pelvic floor, resulting in its weakening over time. Additionally, conditions like continuous coughing, obesity, and hard lifting can further strain the pelvic tissues.

6. Connective Tissue Disorders:
Certain connective tissue illnesses, such as Ehlers-Danlos syndrome, Marfan syndrome, and collagen disorders, can weaken the supportive tissues of the pelvis and elevate the risk of uterine prolapse.

7. Obesity: Excess body weight can place additional stress on the pelvic floor muscles and ligaments, increasing the risk of prolapse. Obesity can also contribute to hormonal imbalances that alter the strength of pelvic tissues.

8. Chronic Respiratory Conditions: Conditions that lead to continuous coughing, such as chronic obstructive pulmonary disease (COPD) or asthma, can exert strain on the pelvic floor and contribute to its weakening.

9. Prior Pelvic Surgery: Certain pelvic surgeries, such as hysterectomy (removal of the uterus), could change the pelvic architecture and weaken the supporting tissues, potentially raising the risk of prolapse.

10. Excessive Physical Activity: Engaging in activities that involve repetitive heavy lifting or intense physical strain might weaken the pelvic floor muscles over time.

11. Age: The risk of uterine prolapse develops with age as the pelvic tissues naturally lose part of their flexibility and power.

12. Ethnic and Cultural Factors: Some research shows that various ethnic and cultural features may influence the occurrence of uterine prolapse. This can be attributable to genetic differences, cultural norms during labour, and lifestyle variables particular to certain ethnicities.

13. Hormonal Changes During Pregnancy: Pregnancy leads to hormonal changes that could affect the connective tissues and muscles of the pelvis. Hormonal fluctuations, particularly the surge in relaxing hormone during pregnancy, might contribute to the weakening of pelvic tissues.

14. Poor Muscle Tone: Inactivity and a sedentary lifestyle can contribute to low muscle tone in the pelvic floor muscles. Weak muscles are less effective at supporting the pelvic organs, increasing the risk of prolapse.

15. Chronic Medical Conditions: Certain chronic medical problems, such as diabetes and chronic renal disease, could influence the overall health of pelvic tissues and lead to the development of uterine prolapse.

16. Heavy Lifting and Occupational Factors: Women who habitually participate in heavy lifting as part of their profession or lifestyle may encounter more strain on the pelvic floor muscles, thereby leading to their weakening and the risk of prolapse.

17. Smoking: Smoking has been related with reduced blood flow to the pelvic area, which can impair the health and strength of pelvic tissues.

18. Poor Posture: Consistently improper posture, especially sitting or standing with severe forward pelvic tilt, can impact the alignment of the pelvic tissues and contribute to prolapse.

19. Lack of Oestrogen Replacement Therapy: In postmenopausal women, the reduction in oestrogen levels could damage pelvic tissues. Hormone replacement treatment (HRT) can assist maintain the health of these tissues and potentially lessen the possibility of prolapse.

20. Multiple Pregnancies and Spacing: Having several pregnancies in a short period without proper recovery time for the pelvic floor muscles to develop strength can increase the risk of uterine prolapse.

21. Lack of Antenatal and Postnatal Care: Inadequate prenatal and postnatal care, including lack of guidance on pelvic floor exercises and postpartum therapy, can contribute to impaired pelvic floor muscles and ligaments.

Understanding the delicate interplay of these factors can enable women to make informed decisions about their health and minimise their risk of uterine prolapse.

If you fear you may be at risk for uterine prolapse or are having symptoms, receiving a medical assessment is crucial. A healthcare provider can analyse your particular risk factors and provide information on applicable preventive steps and treatment possibilities.

Chapter 2

SYMPTOMS OF UTERINE PROLAPSE

Uterine prolapse is a complex disorder that can manifest with a wide range of symptoms, changing in kind and severity based on the degree of prolapse and the structures affected.

These symptoms can impact a woman's physical comfort, emotional well-being, and general quality of life. Here's a full description of the many symptoms related with uterine prolapse:

1. Vaginal Discomfort and Pressure: Women with uterine prolapse frequently report a sense of pressure or discomfort in the vaginal area. This could range from a modest sensation of fullness to more acute feelings of pressure, heaviness, or even a dragging sensation.

2. Pelvic Discomfort: Pelvic discomfort is a prevalent indication of uterine prolapse. Women could feel a dull ache or heaviness in the lower abdominal and pelvic region, particularly after standing for long periods or participating in intense activities.

3. Visible Protrusion or Bulge: In more advanced cases of uterine prolapse, women may report a palpable protrusion or lump at the vaginal opening. This can be the cervix itself or the uterus expanding into the vaginal canal, resulting in a sense of something coming out of the vagina.

4. Lower Back Pain: Uterine prolapse can cause lower back discomfort due to the increasing tension on the lower back muscles and ligaments when the uterus descends.

5. Urinary Symptoms: Uterine prolapse can impair bladder function, resulting in a spectrum of urinary symptoms:

- <u>Stress Urinary Incontinence:</u> Leakage of urine during actions that increase intra-abdominal pressure, such as coughing, sneezing, laughing, or lifting.

- <u>Urinary Urgency and Frequency:</u> An increased need to urinate suddenly and frequently.

- <u>Difficulty Emptying the Bladder:</u> A perception that the bladder isn't entirely emptied after urinating.

6. Bowel Symptoms: Uterine prolapse can impede bowel function, creating several symptoms pertaining to the rectum and bowel movements:

- <u>Difficulty Emptying the Bowels:</u> A sensation of incomplete bowel evacuation following a bowel movement.

- <u>Constipation:</u> Difficulty passing stools due to changes in pelvic anatomy and bowel function.

- <u>Faecal Incontinence:</u> Loss of control over bowel movements.

7. Pain During Intercourse (Dyspareunia): Women with uterine prolapse may endure pain or discomfort during sexual intercourse due to the changing pelvic anatomy and pressure on neighbouring tissues.

8. Vaginal Bleeding or Discharge: The irritation caused by the prolapsed uterus could lead to spotting or increased vaginal discharge.

9. Emotional Impact: Living with uterine prolapse can have emotional impacts, including feelings of humiliation, aggravation, and a diminished sense of self-esteem due to changes in bodily structure and the impact on daily activities.

10. Reduced Quality of Life: The combination of physical discomfort, urinary and intestinal disorders, sexual difficulties, and emotional anguish can substantially diminish a woman's overall quality of life.

11. Lumbosacral discomfort: Uterine prolapse can contribute to discomfort in the lower back and sacral area due to the changing pelvic position and strain on supporting structures.

12. Bulging Sensation: Women with uterine prolapse may express a sensation of bulging or pressure in the vaginal area, particularly when standing, walking, or doing intense activities.

13. Discomfort While Standing or Walking: Symptoms may escalate when standing or walking for extended durations, as the upright position increases the strain on the pelvic floor muscles and tissues.

14. Discomfort during Long Periods of Sitting: Extended periods of sitting can occasionally worsen symptoms, leading to discomfort, pressure, or a sensation of bulging.

15. Incomplete Emptying Sensation: Some women may feel as though the bladder or rectum hasn't emptied totally after urine or bowel movements due to the altered pelvic anatomy.

16. Frequent Urinary Tract Infections (UTIs): Changes in the pelvic anatomy and issues emptying the bladder completely can boost the risk of urinary tract infections.

17. Haemorrhoids: Uterine prolapse can lead to the creation or worsening of haemorrhoids, creating irritation, itching, and pain in the rectal area.

18. Impact on Physical Activities: Symptoms of uterine prolapse could affect a woman's ability to engage in physical activities she once valued, consequently jeopardising her exercise routine and general fitness.

19. Discomfort with clothes: Tight clothes, especially around the waist and pelvic region, can increase discomfort and pressure associated with uterine prolapse.

20. Impair on Daily Activities: As symptoms worsen, uterine prolapse can impair daily activities such as lifting, bending, and even basic chores like housework or childcare.

21. Sleep Disturbances: Discomfort, pressure, and other symptoms can lead to sleep interruptions, lowering the overall quality of slumber.

22. Impact on Mental Well-being: Living with uterine prolapse can have emotional implications, sometimes leading to worry, despair, and lower self-esteem owing to the physical discomfort and hurdles experienced.

23. The feeling of "Falling Out": Women sometimes describe a sensation as if something is "falling out" of the vagina, which can be particularly noticeable when standing or engaging in activities that increase intra-abdominal pressure.

24. Avoidance of Activities: Due to the discomfort and humiliation associated with symptoms, some women may start avoiding particular activities, which can lead to a reduction in their overall quality of life.

25. Impact on Intimacy and Relationships: Symptoms like discomfort during intercourse and mental anxiety can disrupt intimacy and harm relationships.

The symptoms of uterine prolapse can vary widely based on the degree of prolapse, which refers to how far the uterus has descended into the vaginal canal or outside the vaginal opening.

As the degree of prolapse develops, the symptoms may become more pronounced and significant in a woman's normal life. Here's a full study of how symptoms could differ according on the degree of prolapse:

1. Stage 0: No Prolapse (Asymptomatic):
At this phase, there is no prolapse, and some women may not have any noticeable

symptoms. However, even in the absence of symptoms, pelvic floor exercises and preventive measures are necessary to sustain pelvic health.

2. Stage I: Mild Prolapse (Cystocele):

- <u>Symptoms:</u> Women could have modest symptoms such as a sensation of pressure in the vaginal area, particularly after standing for extended periods. There may be occasional soreness during strenuous exertion.

- <u>Physical Findings:</u> The cervix is still within the vaginal canal, and the uterus is slightly depressed. Some women may feel a slight protrusion in the upper vagina during a pelvic check.

3. Stage II: Moderate Prolapse (Cystocele and Rectocele):

- <u>Symptoms:</u> As the uterus lowers farther, symptoms can become more obvious.

Women may detect increased vaginal pressure, a feeling of something coming out of the vagina, and discomfort during intercourse. urinary and gastrointestinal symptoms, such as stress pee incontinence, and constipation, may also appear.

- <u>Physical Findings:</u> The cervix may stretch into or slightly beyond the vaginal opening. Both the anterior (bladder) and posterior (rectum) walls of the vagina may be affected.

4. Stage III: Severe Prolapse (Procidentia):

- <u>Symptoms:</u> As the uterus descends to a greater extent, symptoms become more intense. Women may have substantial discomfort, pee urgency, frequency, and problems emptying the bladder.

Bowel symptoms, such as problems emptying the bowels and faecal incontinence, could also occur. Sexual intercourse may become more challenging due to discomfort and pressure.

- <u>Physical Findings:</u> The uterus may protrude outside the vaginal opening, but it can still be manually reduced back into the vagina. Both bladder and rectal prolapse are typically present.

5. Stage IV: Complete Prolapse (Procidentia):

- <u>Symptoms:</u> At this mature stage, symptoms are often severe and influential on daily functioning. Women may have prolonged discomfort, problems with urination and bowel motions, and severe emotional suffering. Sexual intercourse may be highly unpleasant or impossible.

- <u>Physical Findings:</u> The uterus, bladder, and rectum are outside the vaginal entrance and cannot be physically lowered. The vaginal tissue may become irritated and ulcerated because to exposure.

Some women may endure minor symptoms even at more advanced stages, while others may have more evident symptoms in early stages due to variances in pelvic architecture, muscle tone, and overall health.

If you suspect you have uterine prolapse or are suffering any symptoms, it's vital to consult a healthcare practitioner. They can perform a full examination, diagnose the degree of prolapse, and provide appropriate treatment options based on your individual circumstances.

Early care can help manage symptoms, promote quality of life, and prevent the progression of uterine prolapse.

Chapter 3

<u>IMPACTS OF UTERINE PROLAPSE</u>

Uterine prolapse can have a considerable effect on a woman's physical, emotional, and social well-being. The extent of these consequences can vary according to the degree of prolapse, the intensity of symptoms, and the individual's overall health. Here's a full review of the potential effects of uterine prolapse:

1. Physical Discomfort and Pain:
Uterine prolapse can lead to many bodily discomforts and misery, including:

- <u>Pelvic pain:</u> Women may endure a persistent sensation of pressure, heaviness, or pain in the pelvic region, limiting their ability to complete routine duties comfortably.

- <u>Lower Back discomfort:</u> The changing pelvic posture and strain on the lower back muscles could lead to prolonged lower back ache.

- <u>Vaginal Discomfort:</u> Some women may feel discomfort, soreness, or a sensation of bulging in the vaginal area.

2. Urinary and Bowel Symptoms:

Uterine prolapse can compromise bladder and bowel function, resulting in symptoms such as:

- <u>Urinary Incontinence:</u> Stress urinary incontinence, where leaking happens during actions like laughing, coughing, or sneezing.

- <u>Urinary Urgency and Frequency:</u> An increased need to urinate suddenly and frequently.

- <u>Difficulty Emptying the Bladder:</u> A perception that the bladder hasn't emptied totally after peeing.

- <u>Bowel Discomfort:</u> Difficulty emptying the intestines fully, constipation, and even faecal incontinence.

3. Sexual Challenges:
Uterine prolapse might affect sexual health and intimacy:

- <u>Painful Intercourse:</u> Discomfort and pressure during sexual intercourse (dyspareunia) can make sexual activity uncomfortable or painful.

- <u>Body Image Concerns:</u> Changes in pelvic anatomy and symptoms may impair a woman's body image and self-confidence, decreasing her comfort level during intercourse.

4. Emotional Impact:

Living with uterine prolapse can lead to a range of emotional challenges:

- <u>Embarrassment:</u> The visible or felt bulge and symptoms like urine spilling can be embarrassing, affecting a woman's self-esteem.

- <u>Irritation:</u> The chronic discomfort and limits in daily duties can lead to irritation and a sense of helplessness.

- <u>Anxiety and sadness:</u> The physical discomfort, influence on lifestyle, and concern about the future could contribute to anxiety and unhappiness.

- <u>Social Isolation:</u> Women may avoid social activities due to pain or fear of symptoms appearing in public contexts.

5. Lifestyle Limitations:

Uterine prolapse can affect a woman's abilities to engage in several activities:

- <u>Exercise Limitations:</u> Physical activities and exercise routines may need to be modified or avoided due to discomfort and worries about exacerbating symptoms.

- <u>Work Challenges:</u> Jobs that entail lengthy standing, hard lifting, or physically demanding responsibilities can become troublesome.

6. Sleep Disturbances:

Persistent discomfort and pain can lead to sleep interruptions, lowering a woman's overall quality of rest and adding to tiredness.

7. Impact on Relationships:

Uterine prolapse can affect relationships in different ways:

- <u>Intimacy difficulties:</u> Sexual problems and emotional distress can limit intimacy and strain relationships.

- <u>Communication:</u> A woman's physical constraints and mental issues may hamper communication with loved ones.

8. Decreased Quality of Life:

Collectively, the physical, emotional, and social ramifications of uterine prolapse can lead to a lower overall quality of life, hurting a woman's ability to enjoy daily activities, relationships, and general well-being.

9. Psychological Effects:

Living with uterine prolapse can bring psychological challenges that may require emotional treatment or counselling to manage stress, worry, and despair.

10. Work and Occupational Challenges:

Uterine prolapse can impair a woman's capacity to execute some employment obligations, specifically those that involve lifting, standing for prolonged periods, or engaging in physically demanding activities. This can result in lower work efficiency, increased absenteeism, and potential career limits.

11. Self-Care Limitations:

The discomfort and physical limits associated with uterine prolapse can make self-care chores, such as personal hygiene and grooming, more challenging.

12. Sleep Disturbances and Fatigue:

Persistent discomfort, pain, and the need for multiple trips to the bathroom during the night can lead to sleep issues. Poor sleep quality can contribute to daily tiredness, reduced concentration, and overall decreased productivity.

13. Economic Impact:

Uterine prolapse may lead to increased medical expenses, including doctor visits, diagnostic tests, treatments, and medicines. Additionally, work-related constraints can hamper a woman's earning potential.

14. Increased Healthcare Utilisation:

The physical and emotional effects of uterine prolapse may result in increased visits to healthcare providers, seeking treatment for symptoms, and managing linked health concerns.

15. Impact on Hobbies and Leisure Activities:

Women with uterine prolapse may find that hobbies and leisure activities they once enjoyed are now uncomfortable or impossible to engage in, resulting in a decreased sense of enjoyment and fulfilment.

16. Impact on Body Image and Self-Esteem:

Changes in pelvic anatomy, visible bulges, and symptoms like urine incontinence can damage a woman's body image and self-esteem. This may influence how she perceives herself and interacts with others.

17. Altered Daily Routine:

The need to manage and adjust to the symptoms of uterine prolapse can disturb a woman's daily routine and lead to greater time spent managing her disease.

18. Impact on Parenting and Caregiving:

For women who are parents or carers, the physical discomfort and limitations associated with uterine prolapse could impair their abilities to care for children, family members, or dependents.

19. Coping Mechanisms and Emotional Resilience:

Living with the effects of uterine prolapse can tax a woman's emotional resilience. Developing effective coping methods, obtaining aid from loved ones, and exploring treatment or support groups might help handle these challenges.

20. Decision-Making Regarding Treatment:

The implications of uterine prolapse can impact a woman's decision-making process regarding treatment possibilities. Factors such as symptom intensity, personal preferences, and general health play a role in therapy decisions.

21. Impact on Overall Well-being:

Collectively, the physical discomfort, emotional anguish, and lifestyle constraints associated with uterine prolapse can have a great effect on a woman's complete well-being, compromising her physical health, mental health, and feelings of satisfaction.

If you're having symptoms or challenges associated with uterine prolapse, addressing your concerns with a healthcare professional can lead to tailored therapies that help control symptoms, promote mental well-being, and enhance your overall quality of life.

Chapter 4

DIAGNOSIS

Uterine prolapse is a medical disease that arises when the pelvic floor muscles and ligaments become weak, allowing the uterus to sink or sag into the vaginal canal.

This condition primarily affects women, especially those who have given birth, undergone numerous pregnancies, experienced menopause, or engaged in activities that create strain on the pelvic region.

Seeking a medical evaluation for uterine prolapse is of crucial importance, as it not only assists in controlling the sickness but also preserves general health and well-being.

One of the primary reasons for receiving medical examination while experiencing uterine prolapse is to properly diagnose the severity of the condition.

Uterine prolapse can range from slight to severe, and only a healthcare professional can identify the amount of the prolapse through a full examination. Proper diagnosis ensures that relevant treatment alternatives are assessed, and any difficulties are managed.

Early discovery and response can prevent the condition from progressing, leading to a better likelihood of successful care.

Furthermore, undergoing a medical checkup for uterine prolapse permits a tailored treatment plan to be established. Each individual's situation is unique, and what works for one person may not be suitable for another.

A healthcare physician might take into account elements such as the patient's age, overall health, lifestyle, and desire for future pregnancies in selecting the optimal course of action. This personalised approach guarantees that the treatment plan matches the patient's individual needs and goals.

Effective therapy of uterine prolapse typically includes a combination of conservative approaches, such as pelvic floor exercises, lifestyle improvements, and the use of supportive devices, as well as surgical alternatives for more severe instances.

A medical evaluation serves to guide these decisions, ensuring that the chosen treatment option is both suitable and successful. It also provides an opportunity for patients to ask questions and acquire a better understanding of their situation, leading to more informed decisions about their health.

Another crucial component of receiving a medical checkup for uterine prolapse is the detection and management of probable repercussions.

Uterine prolapse can lead to a multitude of consequences, including urine incontinence, gastrointestinal disorders, discomfort during sexual intercourse, and psychological distress.

A healthcare specialist can analyse these potential complications and address them alongside the primary ailment. This comprehensive approach to care improves the patient's quality of life and overall well-being.

In addition to physical health difficulties, receiving a medical assessment for uterine prolapse provides major psychological and emotional benefits.

Coping with a prolapse can be stressful, creating worry, humiliation, and a diminished feeling of self-esteem. A healthcare provider can offer support, information, and direction, helping the patient negotiate the emotional components of the condition. This holistic approach to care promotes mental well-being and helps the patient feel empowered in managing their health.

Obtaining a medical evaluation while experiencing uterine prolapse is crucial for precise diagnosis, tailored therapy, complication management, and general well-being.

Early detection and early care can prevent the condition from progressing and greatly boost the patient's quality of life. By prioritising medical evaluation, individuals with uterine prolapse take a proactive step towards protecting their health and securing a better, more comfortable future.

THE DIAGNOSTIC PROCESS

The diagnostic process of uterine prolapse comprises a careful evaluation of a patient's symptoms, medical history, and physical examination, which often includes pelvic exams and, in some instances, imaging studies.

The purpose is to properly examine the degree of the prolapse, rule out other potential illnesses, and identify the most effective treatment option. Here's a full summary of the diagnostic process:

1. Medical History: The primary stage is acquiring information regarding the patient's symptoms, medical history, and any important circumstances that might lead to uterine prolapse.

This involves asking about the presence of symptoms such as pelvic pressure, a sense of "something coming out" of the vagina, urine or bowel issues, sexual pain, and any history of pregnancies, deliveries, or surgeries.

2. Physical Examination:

- <u>Pelvic Exam:</u> A pelvic exam is a critical component of the diagnostic process for uterine prolapse. During the exam, the healthcare professional visually inspects the external genitalia and then inserts a speculum into the vagina to evaluate the vaginal walls, cervix, and the degree of prolapse.

- <u>Cervical Position:</u> The position of the cervix with regard to the vaginal walls is checked. In uterine prolapse, the cervix may be forced downward into the vaginal canal.

- <u>Pelvic Organ Prolapse Quantification (POP-Q) Examination:</u> This standardised method allows healthcare providers to assess and rate the degree of prolapse. It involves the use of reference points to determine the location of the vaginal walls and cervix with regard to the hymen.

3. Imaging Studies:

- <u>Pelvic ultrasonography:</u> Transvaginal ultrasonography is a non-invasive imaging treatment that can produce detailed views of the pelvic organs. It is often conducted to check the pelvic floor, uterine position, and any other irregularities. Ultrasound can help rule out other ailments and provide critical information for therapy planning.

- <u>MRI (Magnetic Resonance Imaging):</u> In more complex cases or when further information is needed, MRI may be indicated. MRI produces detailed cross-sectional scans, offering a thorough view of the pelvic anatomy, including the uterus, bladder, and surrounding tissues.

4. Urodynamic Testing: In circumstances where urinary symptoms are severe, urodynamic testing may be performed. This comprises monitoring bladder and urethral function, and analysing how well the bladder is storing and emptying urine. It can assist uncover any difficulties with pee incontinence or other bladder-related ailments.

5. Assessment of Impact on Daily Life: In addition to the physical examination, the healthcare expert will investigate how the uterine prolapse is impacting the patient's quality of life. This includes discussing the degree of symptoms, the patient's desire for future pregnancies, and any choices for therapy.

6. Collaborative Decision-Making: Based on the findings from the medical history, pelvic exam, imaging studies, and the patient's goals, the healthcare professional will discuss treatment possibilities with the patient. This is a collaborative procedure, and the patient's ideas and concerns are taken into account while deciding on the best course of action.

7. Patient Education: An integral part of the diagnostic procedure is patient education. The healthcare specialist takes the time to explain the diagnosis, the factors contributing to uterine prolapse, the different treatment choices, and the potential dangers and benefits of each technique. This knowledge helps the patient to make informed decisions regarding their therapy, establishing a sense of control and eliminating any concern or misunderstanding.

8. Follow-up and Monitoring: After the diagnosis is established, a strategy for follow-up and monitoring is devised. The frequency of follow-up consultations may vary based on the severity of the prolapse, the chosen treatment strategy, and the patient's response to treatment. Regular monitoring ensures that any changes in symptoms or the effectiveness of treatment are immediately addressed, allowing for adjustments if necessary.

9. Conservative care: In cases when the uterine prolapse is minor or the patient's preferences accord with non-surgical treatments, conservative care may be considered. This can comprise pelvic floor exercises (Kegel exercises), lifestyle improvements (such as weight management and avoiding hard lifting), and the use of pessaries, which are supportive devices implanted in the vagina to lend support to the uterus.

10. Surgical Intervention: If the uterine prolapse is severe or severely affects the patient's quality of life, surgical intervention may be necessary. There are several surgical therapies available, each with its own advantages and considerations. Common surgical procedures for uterine prolapse include hysterectomy (removal of the uterus), uterine suspension (elevating the uterus and attaching it to strong supportive tissues), or restoration of weakened pelvic floor structures.

11. Long-term Care and preventive: After treatment, the healthcare provider underlines the requirement of long-term care and preventative activities. This requires maintaining a healthy lifestyle, practising pelvic floor exercises to strengthen the muscles, and being aware of any symptoms that may imply a recurrence or new concerns.

12. Addressing Psychological and Emotional Aspects: Throughout the diagnosis process and subsequent therapy, healthcare providers acknowledge the potential psychological and emotional implications of uterine prolapse. They offer a supportive environment where patients can communicate their issues and receive advice on coping techniques. Addressing these areas contributes to the overall well-being of the patient.

The diagnosis procedure of uterine prolapse needs a thorough evaluation of the patient's history, physical examination (including pelvic exams), imaging studies, and a collaborative approach to therapeutic decision-making.

Patient education, follow-up, and assessment of both physical and emotional factors play crucial roles in ensuring correct care of uterine prolapse, boosting the patient's quality of life, and promoting overall health and well-being. Seeking medical assessment and engaging in open discussion with healthcare specialists are key factors in resolving this sickness.

Chapter 5

<u>FAMOUS MISCONCEPTIONS</u>

Despite its frequency, there are several common misunderstandings and stigmas surrounding the diagnosis of uterine prolapse. These misunderstandings can lead to disinformation, unwarranted anxiety, and hurdles to accessing competent medical examinations and treatment.

It's crucial to address these beliefs to promote knowledge, minimise stigma, and ensure that women receive the care and help they need. Here are some of the frequent myths and stigmas:

1. It's Rare: One big misunderstanding is that uterine prolapse is a rare ailment. In truth, it's more widespread than many people realise, especially among women who have given birth or have undergone other events that stress the pelvic region. By acknowledging its frequency, we may stress the requirement of adequate assessment and treatment.

2. It's a Normal Component of Aging: While it's true that factors like ageing and hormonal changes can contribute to the weakening of pelvic floor tissues, uterine prolapse is not an inevitable component of getting older. It's a medical issue that can be treated, controlled, and prevented with appropriate therapy, including pelvic floor exercises and, if necessary, surgical operations.

3. It's Caused Only by Childbirth: While childbirth is a considerable risk factor for uterine prolapse, it's not the only cause. Other variables such as repeated pregnancies, persistent coughing, obesity, hard lifting, inherited vulnerability, and hormonal changes around menopause can contribute to the development of uterine prolapse.

4. Surgery is the single answer: Although surgery is an option for severe instances, it's not the entire answer. Mild to severe instances can often be treated by conservative techniques like pelvic floor exercises and the use of supportive devices like pessaries. Early diagnosis and appropriate treatment can prevent the need for surgery in many cases.

5. It's a Sign of Negligence: Some persons incorrectly consider that uterine prolapse is a sign of carelessness or poor self-care. This stigma might lead to emotions of guilt or shame for afflicted folks. However, uterine prolapse is a medical illness influenced by various circumstances, many of which are beyond a person's control.

6. It Only Affects Older Women: While uterine prolapse is more frequent in older women, it can afflict women of all ages, especially those who have undergone acute stress on the pelvic floor. Raising awareness about this issue helps women of all ages recognize the necessity for proper pelvic health.

7. It's Just a Cosmetic Issue: Uterine prolapse is not merely a cosmetic problem; it can have a considerable influence on a woman's quality of life. It may cause discomfort, pain, urinary and bowel problems, sexual difficulties, and even psychological misery. Treating uterine prolapse isn't only about beauty; it's about general health and well-being.

8. It Can't Be Prevented: While certain risk factors for uterine prolapse, such as heredity, can't be changed, there are preventive activities that can lower the likelihood of acquiring the disease.

Maintaining a healthy weight, exercising pelvic floor exercises, avoiding excessive lifting, and effectively managing chronic conditions that lead to coughing can all contribute to prevention.

9. It's Not a Valid issue: Some folks may dismiss the relevance of uterine prolapse, considering it a petty issue. However, the symptoms and influence on daily functioning can be severe. Acknowledging these difficulties is crucial for delivering effective care and aid to impacted folks.

10. It's Embarrassing to Talk About: Due to the stigma surrounding pelvic health and reproductive concerns, some women may feel ashamed to discuss uterine prolapse with healthcare practitioners or even with family and friends. Open communication is crucial for appropriate diagnosis, treatment, and emotional support. Healthcare practitioners are taught to handle these interactions with respect and empathy.

11. It's a Sign of Weakness: Some folks may wrongly interpret uterine prolapse as a sign of personal weakness or a lack of perseverance. This misunderstanding could lead to emotions of self-blame for those suffering from the condition. It's crucial to recognize that uterine prolapse is a complex medical issue influenced by a range of circumstances, many of which are beyond an individual's control. It is not a reflection of personal character or strength.

12. It's Not significant Enough to Seek Medical Attention: Some women might downplay their symptoms or delay seeking medical examination because they feel uterine prolapse isn't significant enough. However, even mild cases of uterine prolapse can lead to discomfort, disruption of regular activities, and impair general well-being. Early detection and effective medication are crucial to prevent the worsening of the condition and its probable ramifications.

13. It Only Affects Women Who Have Given Birth: While delivery is a big risk factor, uterine prolapse can occur in women who haven't had children. Other variables, like frequent coughing, obesity, and inherited vulnerability, might contribute to the weakening of pelvic floor muscles and ligaments. Understanding the whole range of risk factors helps ensure that all patients at risk receive appropriate care.

14. It's a Private Matter and Shouldn't Be Discussed Publicly: The stigma surrounding pelvic health issues sometimes contributes to the idea that these matters should stay private. While it's vital to respect an individual's privacy and comfort level, fostering open discussions about uterine prolapse is critical for raising awareness, lowering stigma, and delivering valuable information to those in need. Public conversation can lead to improved understanding and more educated decisions concerning pelvic health.

15. Treatment is Not Worth the Effort: Some women may feel overwhelmed by the treatment options or assume that treating uterine prolapse isn't worth the effort. However, treatment can greatly enhance the quality of life, alleviate symptoms, and avert consequences. It's vital to review treatment possibilities with a healthcare practitioner and consider the prospective benefits in terms of general well-being.

16. It Can't Impact Sexual Health: Uterine prolapse can impair sexual health in different ways. Discomfort, pain, or changes in the anatomy of the pelvic area may contribute to sexual difficulties. Addressing these issues with healthcare experts is vital to guarantee that sexual health and intimacy are not overlooked.

17. It Can't recur After Treatment:
While good treatment can give comfort and improve symptoms, it's vital to be aware that uterine prolapse can recur, especially if risk factors are not addressed. Regular follow-up sessions and attention to preventive measures are important to monitor for recurrence and preserve pelvic health.

By refuting these popular misunderstandings and breaking down the stigma surrounding uterine prolapse, we can create a more informed and supportive culture for women suffering from this disease.

Education, open communication, and a caring attitude to healthcare can make a tremendous difference in helping women receive the appropriate care, control their symptoms, and lead healthier, more happy lives.

Chapter 6

<u>CONSERVATIVE THERAPY APPROACHES</u>

Conservative therapy techniques for uterine prolapse are generally the initial line of treatments, particularly in cases of mild to moderate prolapse or when surgical intervention is not immediately necessary or requested by the patient.

These procedures try to reduce symptoms, increase pelvic support, and enhance the patient's general quality of life without the need for surgery.

They may comprise a combination of lifestyle improvements, pelvic floor exercises, the use of supporting devices, and regular follow-up to assess progress. Here's a full summary of conservative therapy options:

Pelvic Floor Exercises (Kegel Exercises)

Strengthening the pelvic floor muscles is a critical feature of conservative management. These exercises, often known as Kegel exercises, involve contracting and relaxing the muscles that support the pelvic organs.

A healthcare professional or a pelvic floor physical therapist can advise the patient on how to conduct these exercises efficiently. Consistent and effective Kegel exercises can boost pelvic muscle tone and assist maintain the uterus, lessening the symptoms of prolapse.

Lifestyle Modifications

- <u>Weight Management:</u> Excess weight can exert additional strain on the pelvic floor, exacerbating prolapse symptoms. Maintaining a healthy weight with a balanced diet and regular exercise helps lessen this pressure and provide pelvic support.

- <u>Dietary Changes:</u> A diet heavy in fibre can minimise constipation, which can strain the pelvic floor. Adequate water and a diet focused on natural foods can contribute to overall gut health.

- <u>Avoiding hard Lifting:</u> Reducing hard lifting or adopting suitable lifting techniques can lessen pressure on the pelvic region and assist prevent future prolapse.

Supportive Devices (Pessaries)

Pessaries are medical devices used to supply support to the pelvic organs and alleviate prolapse symptoms. These are placed into the vagina to assist raise the uterus and support the surrounding structures.

Pessaries vary in numerous forms and sizes, and a healthcare specialist could advise the most suitable variety based on the patient's individual situation.

Biofeedback and Physical Therapy

In rare cases, biofeedback techniques can be utilised to increase pelvic muscle synchrony during activities. Physical therapists with expertise in pelvic floor rehabilitation can provide useful assistance and therapies to strengthen and maintain the pelvic floor.

Hormone Therapy

For postmenopausal women, hormone replacement therapy (HRT) may be explored. Oestrogen therapy can increase the flexibility and strength of pelvic tissues, potentially lessening prolapse symptoms. However, the usage of HRT should be discussed with a healthcare provider, considering the patient's general health and individual circumstances.

Regular Follow-up

Monitoring the success of conservative treatment is crucial. Patients should have regular follow-up visits with their healthcare practitioner to evaluate progress, discuss any concerns, and make needed adjustments to the treatment plan.

Educational and Emotional Support

Offering education and emotional support to patients is vital. This includes discussing the condition, its causes, treatment possibilities, projected consequences, and addressing any emotional anxieties or misconceptions that the patient may have. Creating an environment where patients may openly communicate their experiences helps establish trust and encourages treatment adherence.

Pain Management

If discomfort or pain is a major problem, non-prescription pain medications or anti-inflammatory drugs may be prescribed to assist manage symptoms.

Prolapse-Specific Physical Activities

Healthcare practitioners can advise patients on activities that might worsen prolapse symptoms and provide ideas on other workouts or adjustments that are less likely to strain the pelvic floor.

Behavioural Changes

Healthcare experts can assist patients realise the requirement of avoiding habits that could trigger prolapse, such as straining during bowel movements or holding one's breath while heavy lifting.

Posture Awareness

Proper posture can play a role in decreasing intra-abdominal pressure and minimising strain on the pelvic floor. Healthcare providers can educate patients on maintaining appropriate posture throughout regular activities.

Cleanliness and Self-Care

Proper cleaning and self-care are key elements of controlling uterine prolapse. Patients should be taught on maintaining adequate vaginal hygiene to prevent infections and pain. Additionally, healthcare experts can explain strategies to lessen the impact of prolapse on daily activities, such as avoiding prolonged standing or sitting, adopting excellent body mechanics, and taking breaks when needed.

Education on Symptoms and Monitoring

Patients should be informed about the symptoms of uterine prolapse and how to spot any changes or worsening of the sickness. Monitoring symptoms and discussing any concerns with a healthcare practitioner can lead to early alterations in the treatment plan and improved overall management.

Preventing or Managing Constipation

Constipation can strain the pelvic floor and worsen prolapse symptoms. Healthcare specialists can provide advice on keeping regular bowel movements through dietary modifications, optimum hydration, and suitable toileting habits. In some instances, the use of stool softeners or laxatives could be advised.

Addressing Urinary Concerns

If urinary incontinence or other pee symptoms are present, healthcare experts can suggest ways for controlling these challenges. This may include bladder training, scheduled voiding, and steps to restrict fluid intake before night.

Exploring Relaxation Techniques

Chronic muscle tension might exacerbate pelvic floor issues. Healthcare specialists may provide relaxation strategies, such as deep breathing, gentle stretching, or practices like yoga, to assist reduce muscle tension and promote general well-being.

Support Groups and therapy

For patients feeling mental discomfort or wanting more support, joining in support groups or seeking therapy could be beneficial. Sharing experiences with others who understand the challenge of living with prolapse might make people feel less alienated and more strong in controlling their disease.

Long-Term Care and Prevention

Even after effective therapy of uterine prolapse, long-term care and preventive measures are needed. Patients should be instructed about the need of continuing pelvic floor exercises, having a healthy lifestyle, and being aware of any changes that would need further evaluation.

Regular Gynecological Check-ups

Regular gynaecological check-ups are necessary for monitoring the disease, especially if the patient's symptoms persist or fluctuate. These check-ups allow healthcare experts to examine the progress of conservative treatment, address any new concerns, and determine if adjustments to the treatment plan are required.

Individualised Approach

It's vital to note that every patient's experience with uterine prolapse is unique. A tailored approach to treatment is vital to address particular needs, preferences, and health conditions. Healthcare practitioners should take the time to grasp the patient's circumstances fully and cooperate on a treatment plan that meets the patient's goals and general well-being.

By emphasising conservative treatment options and giving comprehensive care that addresses physical, emotional, and educational requirements, healthcare practitioners can enable patients to actively participate in treating uterine prolapse. This technique not only improves symptom management but also promotes overall pelvic health, enables patients to make educated decisions, and aids to a better quality of life for people suffering from this disease.

Chapter 7

<u>MEDICAL AND SURGICAL</u> <u>INTERVENTIONS</u>

Medical and surgical procedures for uterine prolapse are meant to address more severe instances where conservative therapies may not deliver significant relief or when the prolapse severely impairs the patient's quality of life.

These interventions try to restore pelvic support, reduce symptoms, and improve the overall pelvic health of the patient. The decision to intervene depends on various aspects, including the severity of the prolapse, the patient's overall health, their desire for future pregnancies, and individual preferences. Here's a full description of pharmacological and surgical therapy options:

HORMONE REPLACEMENT THERAPY (HRT)

For postmenopausal women, hormone replacement therapy can be considered to increase the flexibility and strength of pelvic tissues, potentially lessening prolapse symptoms. However, the usage of HRT should be discussed with a healthcare provider, considering the patient's general health and individual circumstances.

Benefits of Hormone Replacement Therapy (HRT) for Uterine Prolapse

1. <u>Improved Pelvic Tissue Health:</u> HRT, particularly oestrogen therapy, can help boost the health and elasticity of pelvic tissues, including the vaginal walls and supporting structures. This can be useful for women experiencing thinning and weakening of these tissues owing to hormonal changes, such as those that occur after menopause.

2. <u>Reduced Vaginal Dryness:</u> Oestrogen therapy can reduce vaginal dryness, making sexual intercourse more comfortable and lowering discomfort or pain associated with vaginal dryness.

3. <u>Potential for Symptom Relief:</u> Some women with uterine prolapse may endure discomfort or anguish related to the condition, particularly if the tissues grow more fragile or less elastic. HRT might help reduce some of these symptoms by maintaining tissue health.

4. <u>Preservation of Pelvic Support:</u> Oestrogen therapy may help maintain the strength and resilience of pelvic tissues, potentially providing greater support to the pelvic organs, including the uterus.

5. <u>Non-Surgical Option:</u> For women who prefer to avoid surgical procedures or who may not be suitable candidates for surgery, HRT provides a non-surgical option to

manage some of the symptoms and tissue changes associated with uterine prolapse.

Risks of Hormone Replacement Therapy (HRT) for Uterine Prolapse

1. <u>Increased Risk of Certain Health Conditions:</u> Long-term use of hormone replacement therapy, especially systemic oestrogen therapy, has been associated with an increased risk of certain health conditions, including cardiovascular disease, stroke, blood clots, and certain types of cancer (such as breast cancer and endometrial cancer). The overall risk relies on factors such as age, duration of therapy, and individual health history.

2. <u>Breast pain and Swelling:</u> Some women may develop breast soreness or swelling as a side effect of HRT.

3. <u>Irregular Bleeding:</u> Oestrogen medication, especially when taken with

progesterone, can lead to irregular bleeding or spotting, particularly in women who still have their uterus.

4. <u>Gallbladder Issues:</u> There may be a slightly increased risk of gallbladder sickness related to HRT.

5. <u>Changes in Mood or Emotional Well-being:</u> Hormone changes can alter mood and emotional well-being in some women. This may involve symptoms such as mood swings, anger, or even depression symptoms.

6. <u>Individual Variation:</u> Not all women will experience the same advantages or hazards with HRT. Individual responses to hormone therapy can vary, and some women may have more considerable alleviation from symptoms while others may not.

7. <u>Interaction with Other Medications:</u> HRT may interact with other medications the

individual is taking, hence it's crucial to examine potential interactions with a healthcare specialist.

PESSARY

A pessary, a medical device, can be used as a non-surgical technique to supply support to the uterus and relieve discomfort. It's a detachable item that is placed into the vagina.

Pessaries vary in numerous forms and sizes, and a healthcare specialist could advise the most suitable variety based on the patient's individual situation. Pessaries are particularly beneficial for women who desire a non-surgical technique or those who are not acceptable candidates for surgery.

Benefits of Pessary for Uterine Prolapse

1. <u>Non-Invasive technique:</u> Pessary insertion is a non-invasive technique to manage

uterine prolapse, making it an attractive alternative for women who prefer to avoid surgery or who may not be ideal candidates for surgery owing to medical concerns.

2. <u>Preserves Fertility:</u> For women who wish to have additional children, a pessary can be an excellent way to manage prolapse while protecting fertility. Surgical interventions may limit future childbearing.

3. <u>Customizable:</u> Pessaries come in many shapes and sizes, allowing healthcare personnel to choose the most suitable solution for each patient. This change enhances comfort and efficacy.

4. <u>Improves Quality of Life:</u> Properly fitted pessaries can considerably reduce the symptoms of uterine prolapse, such as pelvic pressure, vaginal discomfort, and urine issues, leading to a higher quality of life.

5. <u>Reversible:</u> Pessaries can be removed at any moment by a healthcare practitioner. If a woman develops pain or decides to explore other treatment options, the pessary can be simply removed without permanent alterations.

6. <u>Avoids General Anesthesia:</u> Unlike surgical therapies, pessary installation does not require general anaesthesia, which might have its own set of hazards.

<u>Risks and Considerations of Pessary Use</u>

1. <u>Pessary Fitting Issues:</u> The success of a pessary depends on good fitting by a qualified healthcare provider. An ill-fitted pessary may not supply the appropriate support and may generate discomfort or complications.

2. <u>Chance of Infection:</u> Pessaries need frequent cleaning and care to decrease the chance of infection. In some conditions,

women may be prone to urinary tract infections or vaginal infections due to the presence of the pessary.

3. <u>Discomfort or anguish:</u> While many women find relief with a well-fitted pessary, some may endure discomfort or misery, especially during the adjustment period. This discomfort can frequently be alleviated with modifications to the type or size of the pessary.

4. <u>Expulsion:</u> In some instances, the pessary may fall out of place or be evacuated by the body. This necessitates quick attention from a healthcare provider to resolve the condition.

5. <u>Monitoring:</u> Regular follow-up visits with a healthcare practitioner are crucial to check the pessary's effectiveness, resolve any issues, and ensure that it remains in the correct spot.

6.   <u>Potential   Interference   with   Sexual Activity:</u> Depending on the type of pessary and individual anatomy, some women may realise that the presence of the pessary hinders sexual activity or causes discomfort during intercourse.

7. <u>Long-Term Use:</u> If a pessary is chosen as a long-term alternative, it may require continuous maintenance and replacements, which can be difficult for some women.

It's vital for women considering a pessary for uterine prolapse to discuss the benefits, risks, and alternatives with their healthcare specialists.

Each woman's health is unique, and a complete evaluation is vital to determine the most effective treatment plan that corresponds with her medical history, goals, and preferences.

TOPICAL OESTROGEN THERAPY

For women who are not candidates for systemic hormone therapy, topical oestrogen creams or vaginal suppositories can be provided. These localised therapies can help promote the health and flexibility of vaginal tissues, which may reduce some of the symptoms associated with uterine prolapse.

Topical oestrogen therapy is a technique of hormone replacement therapy (HRT) that involves applying oestrogen-containing creams, gels, or vaginal rings directly to the vaginal tissues.

This treatment is primarily used to address complaints of vaginal atrophy and urogenital issues in postmenopausal women, but it can also have potential benefits and hazards when considered as a therapeutic option for uterine prolapse. Let's evaluate the benefits and dangers of topical oestrogen therapy specifically for uterine prolapse:

Benefits of Topical Oestrogen Therapy for Uterine Prolapse

1. <u>Tissue Health:</u> Oestrogen is a hormone that performs a key function in maintaining the health of the vaginal and pelvic tissues. Topical oestrogen therapy can assist boost the flexibility, thickness, and overall health of the vaginal tissues, which may indirectly aid individuals with uterine prolapse.

2. <u>Vaginal Lubrication:</u> Oestrogen therapy can help decrease vaginal dryness, making sexual intercourse more comfortable for women experiencing vaginal atrophy due to hormonal changes, which can be particularly helpful for women with uterine prolapse who may experience discomfort during sexual activity.

3. <u>Support for Pelvic Muscles:</u> Some studies suggest that oestrogen therapy may

contribute to the maintenance of pelvic muscle strength and function, which can potentially have a favourable impact on pelvic organ support, including the uterus.

4. <u>Complementary Therapy:</u> Topical oestrogen therapy can be used as a complementary strategy alongside other non-surgical treatments for uterine prolapse, such as pelvic floor exercises or the use of pessaries. It may increase the effectiveness of these drugs.

5. <u>Minimal Systemic Effects:</u> Unlike systemic oestrogen therapy, which involves taking oestrogen orally or through other systemic routes, topical oestrogen therapy has less systemic effects. This tailored dosing decreases the chance of systemic side effects such as blood clots, stroke, and breast cancer.

6. <u>Preservation of Uterine Tissues:</u> For women who prefer to keep their uterine

tissues, topical oestrogen therapy may give a non-surgical option to maintain uterine health.

<u>Risks and Considerations of Topical Oestrogen Therapy for Uterine Prolapse</u>

1. <u>Limited impact on Prolapse:</u> While oestrogen therapy can improve vaginal health, it may not dramatically alter the physical support of the uterus or halt its descent. It is primarily effective for alleviating vaginal atrophy and urogenital symptoms rather than providing mechanical support for uterine prolapse.

2. <u>Individual Response:</u> Not all women will obtain the same degree of benefit from topical oestrogen therapy. Individual responses to oestrogen treatment can vary, and some women may obtain minimal improvement from their uterine prolapse symptoms.

3. <u>Potential undesirable Effects:</u> Although topical oestrogen therapy has fewer systemic effects than systemic HRT, there are still potential adverse effects, including localised discomfort, itching, or discharge in the vaginal area. These unpleasant effects are usually temporary and can be treated.

4. <u>Monitoring and Follow-up:</u> Women undergoing topical oestrogen therapy should have regular follow-up consultations with their healthcare provider to monitor the therapy's effectiveness and discuss any conccrns.

5. <u>Breast Cancer Concerns:</u> Although the risk of breast cancer connected with topical oestrogen therapy is considered lower than with systemic HRT, women with a history of breast cancer or those at higher risk should discuss this potential risk with their healthcare professional.

6. <u>Alternative Treatments:</u> While topical oestrogen therapy can deliver some benefits for vaginal health, it may not be the most effective sole treatment for uterine prolapse, especially in more severe cases. Women with severe uterine prolapse may need to consider other treatment options, such as pessaries or surgical surgery, to address the underlying issue.

Topical oestrogen therapy can offer benefits for vaginal health and may have a supportive role in resolving uterine prolapse symptoms, especially when accompanied with other non-surgical treatments.

However, it's vital for women to have a lengthy chat with their healthcare professional about the potential benefits, hazards, and alternatives for their individual circumstance. A personalised strategy, analysing the severity of the uterine prolapse and specific health issues, is important to pick the most matched treatment plan.

UTERINE SUSPENSION (SACRAL COLPOPEXY)

This surgical approach comprises attaching the uterus to strong supporting structures in the pelvic region, effectively restoring it to a more anatomically normal position. This procedure gives long-term support and stability, making it a common surgical choice for women who choose to maintain their uterus, especially if more pregnancies are desired.

Benefits of Uterine Suspension (Sacral Colpopexy) for Uterine Prolapse

1. Effective Correction: Sacral colpopexy is a highly effective operation for repairing uterine prolapse, especially in circumstances of severe prolapse where alternative

non-surgical treatments may be less successful.

2. <u>Long-Term Relief: When</u> effective, sacral colpopexy can provide long-term relief from the symptoms of uterine prolapse, including pelvic pressure, discomfort, urinary issues, and difficulty with bowel movements.

3. <u>Restoration of Normal Anatomy:</u> The procedure seeks to return the uterus to its proper anatomical position within the pelvis, which can reduce both functional and aesthetic concerns associated with prolapse.

4. <u>Improved Quality of Life:</u> Many women report a considerable boost in their quality of life after sacral colpopexy, as the surgery resolves the underlying issue of uterine descent, allowing them to resume normal activities without discomfort or limits.

5. <u>Preservation of Uterus:</u> In instances when the lady decides to save her uterus for

personal or medical reasons, sacral colpopexy presents an alternative to correct prolapse while retaining the uterus.

6. <u>Potential for Concurrent Procedures:</u> Sacral colpopexy can be combined with other pelvic floor repairs or procedures, such as bladder or rectal prolapse repair, to comprehensively address numerous problems during a single surgery.

Risks and Considerations of Uterine Suspension (Sacral Colpopexy)

1. <u>Surgical Risks:</u> As with any surgical surgery, sacral colpopexy includes intrinsic surgical risks, such as infection, bleeding, anaesthesia issues, and adverse responses to medicines.

2. <u>Recovery phase:</u> The recovery phase following sacral colpopexy can be several weeks, during which the patient may feel discomfort, limited physical activity, and limits on carrying heavy objects. This

healing period should be properly planned and handled with the surgeon.

3. <u>Potential for Recurrence:</u> Although sacral colpopexy has a high success rate, there is a minor risk of recurrence of prolapse over time. Regular follow-up consultations with the surgeon are essential to examine the long-term consequences of the procedure.

4. <u>Postoperative Complications:</u> There can be complications particular to the surgery, such as mesh-related issues (if the mesh is employed), injury to surrounding structures, or concerns linked to the sutures or fixation materials used to maintain the uterus.

5. <u>Anaesthesia hazards:</u> Anesthesia brings its own set of concerns, including reactions, breathing difficulties, or uncommon but serious complications.

6. <u>Loss of Uterus:</u> For certain ladies, the removal of the uterus (hysterectomy) may

be needed following sacral colpopexy, especially if the uterus is substantially affected or if the lady wishes to avoid future prolapse difficulties.

7. <u>Personal Considerations:</u> The decision to have sacral colpopexy should be chosen by the individual's medical history, overall health, desire for future pregnancies (because it may reduce fertility), and personal preferences.

It's crucial for women considering sacrocolpopexy for uterine prolapse to have a lengthy chat with their healthcare practitioner and a qualified surgeon. The decision should be reached based on a complete examination of the specific case, assessing the benefits against the potential hazards, and taking into account the woman's overall health and preferences.

HYSTERECTOMY

In cases where the patient does not desire to preserve the uterus or when other therapies are not helpful, a hysterectomy may be indicated. This surgical method involves the removal of the uterus.

It can be performed via traditional open surgery, laparoscopic methods, or minimally invasive robotic-assisted surgery. A hysterectomy can effectively address uterine prolapse and may be coupled with additional procedures, such as rebuilding the pelvic floor.

Hysterectomy is a surgical surgery that involves the removal of the uterus, and in certain situations, the cervix. It is a final therapeutic option for uterine prolapse, a disease where the uterus descends or alters from its natural place within the pelvis.

While a hysterectomy can effectively repair uterine prolapse, it's crucial to understand the benefits and dangers related with this procedure before making a decision. Let's review the benefits and risks of hysterectomy for uterine prolapse in detail:

Benefits of Hysterectomy for Uterine Prolapse

1. <u>Permanent cure:</u> Hysterectomy is a proven remedy for uterine prolapse. Once the uterus is removed, the risk of future prolapse is eliminated, and the patient will no longer have symptoms linked to uterine prolapse.

2. <u>Relief from Symptoms:</u> Hysterectomy can alleviate the symptoms associated with uterine prolapse, such as pelvic pressure, discomfort, urination issues, bowel problems, and vaginal bulging. Many ladies obtain substantial respite from these difficulties following the treatment.

3. <u>Improved Quality of Life:</u> For women whose quality of life is substantially impacted by uterine prolapse, a successful

hysterectomy can lead to a marked boost in overall well-being, allowing them to resume normal activities without the constraints imposed by prolapse-related symptoms.

4. <u>Treatment of Concurrent Conditions:</u> If a woman has other medical conditions that can be addressed through a hysterectomy, such as uterine fibroids, abnormal bleeding, or certain types of gynecologic cancers, a hysterectomy can serve as a comprehensive treatment option, simultaneously addressing these conditions along with uterine prolapse.

5. <u>Potential for Combined Procedures:</u> If needed, a hysterectomy can be combined with additional pelvic floor repairs or operations, such as bladder or rectal prolapse repair or incontinence procedures, to address numerous diseases during a single surgery.

Risks and Considerations of Hysterectomy for Uterine Prolapse

1. <u>Surgical Risks:</u> Like any surgical treatment, a hysterectomy includes inherent surgical risks, including infection, bleeding, unpleasant responses to anaesthesia or medicines, injury to adjacent structures, and the probability of postoperative difficulties.

2. <u>Recovery Period:</u> Recovery following a hysterectomy can take several weeks, and during this time, the patient may suffer pain, limited physical activity, and limits on lifting heavy objects. The recuperation length should be thoroughly discussed with the surgeon.

3. <u>Loss of Fertility:</u> A hysterectomy results in the permanent loss of fertility, making it a significant option for women who still wish to have children. This decision should be done in consultation with the healthcare expert, considering the woman's age, family planning goals, and other considerations.

4. <u>Hormonal Changes:</u> In cases where the ovaries are removed combined with the uterus (a treatment known as bilateral salpingo-oophorectomy), there might be hormonal changes that may lead to menopause, potentially creating symptoms such as hot flashes, mood disorders, and other menopausal symptoms.

5. <u>Long-Term Health Considerations:</u> Some studies suggest that hysterectomy may be related with a slightly greater risk of certain health issues, such as cardiovascular disease and bone density abnormalities. However, the extent of this risk and the impact of other factors remain matters of continuous inquiry.

6. <u>Potential Impact on Sexual Function:</u> While many women do not report dramatic changes in sexual function after a hysterectomy, some may have worries about how the procedure might influence their

sexual experience. Open engagement with the healthcare practitioner about such concerns is crucial.

7.   <u>Psychological Considerations:</u> A hysterectomy is a substantial medical treatment that involves the removal of a reproductive organ. Some women may endure emotional or psychological ramifications linked with the loss of the uterus, and these feelings should be addressed and handled.

8.   <u>Alternative Treatments:</u> In certain instances, less invasive or non-surgical treatments, such as pelvic floor exercises, pessaries, or topical oestrogen therapy, may be useful in treating uterine prolapse without the need for a hysterectomy.

It's essential for women considering a hysterectomy for uterine prolapse to have a comprehensive discussion with their healthcare provider, ideally with a gynaecologist or urogynecologist, to carefully weigh the benefits, risks, and alternatives based on their individual medical history, overall health, family planning goals, and personal preferences. A personalised strategy that takes into consideration the unique conditions is crucial to make an informed conclusion.

ANTERIOR AND POSTERIOR REPAIR (COLPORRHAPHY)

This surgical treatment tries to mend the front (anterior) and rear (posterior) vaginal walls, which may be weakened or bulging as a result of uterine prolapse. The surgeon tightens and reinforces these tissues, repairing the prolapse and restoring support to the pelvic organs.

Anterior and posterior repair, commonly known as colporrhaphy, are surgical methods that address distinct types of pelvic organ prolapse. These treatments are conducted to repair the front (anterior) and rear (posterior) vaginal walls when they have deteriorated or declined due to uterine prolapse.

Anterior repair tackles a cystocele, which is the prolapse of the bladder into the vaginal wall, while posterior repair addresses a rectocele, which is the prolapse of the rectum into the vaginal wall. Let's analyse the benefits and concerns of anterior and posterior repair (colporrhaphy) for uterine prolapse:

Benefits of Anterior and Posterior Repair (Colporrhaphy) for Uterine Prolapse

1. <u>Targeted Correction:</u> Anterior and posterior repair specifically target the prolapsed sections of the vaginal walls, giving exact correction for the damaged compartments. This concentrated method can significantly alleviate symptoms linked with cystocele or rectocele.

2.   <u>Relief from Pelvic Symptoms:</u> Colporrhaphy can alleviate symptoms such as pelvic pressure, vaginal bulging, discomfort, and trouble with urine or bowel function that often accompany uterine prolapse.

3. <u>Improved Quality of Life:</u> Many women find a significant rise in their quality of life after successful anterior or posterior surgery, allowing them to resume regular activities without the limits imposed by prolapse-related symptoms.

4. <u>Minimally Invasive Options:</u> Depending on the severity of the prolapse and the surgical approach chosen by the healthcare provider, anterior and posterior repair can often be performed using minimally invasive techniques, such as laparoscopic or robotic-assisted surgery, leading to shorter hospital stays, less postoperative pain, and

faster recovery compared to traditional open surgery.

5. <u>Preservation of Uterus:</u> Anterior and posterior repair therapies allow women who choose to preserve their uterus to avoid a hysterectomy, as these operations focus on the vaginal wall support rather than removal of the uterus.

6. <u>Potential for Combined Procedures:</u> If needed, an anterior or posterior repair can be combined with further pelvic floor repairs or surgeries to address numerous issues during a single procedure, allowing full treatment for difficult situations.

<u>Risks and Considerations of Anterior and Posterior Repair (Colporrhaphy) for Uterine Prolapse</u>

1. <u>Surgical Risks:</u> Like any surgical operation, colporrhaphy contains inherent surgical risks, including infection, bleeding, unpleasant responses to anaesthesia or

medicines, injury to neighbouring structures, and the potential of postoperative difficulties.

2. <u>Recurrence:</u> While colporrhaphy helps provide short-term comfort, there is a slight probability of recurrence of prolapse over time. Regular follow-up consultations with the surgeon are essential to examine the long-term consequences of the procedure.

3. <u>Recovery Period:</u> Recovery from colporrhaphy could take several weeks, during which the patient may endure pain, limited physical activity, and restrictions on carrying heavy objects. The recuperation length should be thoroughly discussed with the surgeon.

4. <u>Potential for Future Prolapse:</u> It's crucial to recognize that colporrhaphy targets the specific compartments involved in uterine prolapse, but it doesn't preclude the

possibility of prolapse emerging in additional compartments in the future.

5. <u>Alternative Treatments:</u> In certain instances, additional non-surgical treatments, such pelvic floor exercises, pessaries, or topical oestrogen therapy, may be useful in managing uterine prolapse without the need for surgical intervention.

The choice to proceed with colporrhaphy should be based on a complete examination of the unique circumstances, assessing the benefits against the potential hazards, and taking into account the woman's overall health, surgical history, and personal preferences.

6. <u>Hormonal difficulties:</u> If a woman has undergone a hysterectomy along with anterior and/or posterior repair, there may be hormonal issues if the ovaries were removed (bilateral salpingo-oophorectomy),

which can lead to menopause and its associated symptoms.

It's crucial for women seeking anterior and posterior repair (colporrhaphy) for uterine prolapse to have a detailed talk with their healthcare professional, ideally with a gynaecologist or urogynecologist.

This consultation should thoroughly explore the benefits, hazards, and alternatives based on their individual medical history, overall health, family planning goals, and personal preferences.

A personalised strategy that takes into consideration the unique conditions is crucial to making an informed selection regarding the most suitable treatment option.

COMBINATION OF TECHNIQUES

Depending on the particular conditions and the severity of prolapse, a variety of surgical treatments may be indicated. For example, a hysterectomy may be coupled with other treatments to manage prolapse and mend weakened pelvic tissues.

A combination of procedures, often referred to as a "prolapse repair surgery" or "pelvic organ prolapse (POP) repair," involves the simultaneous or staged repair of multiple pelvic organ prolapses, which may include uterine prolapse along with other prolapsed structures such as the bladder (cystocele) or rectum (rectocele).

This approach tries to comprehensively address the myriad prolapse difficulties a lady may be suffering. The decision to conduct a combination of surgeries should be carefully reviewed, taking into account the benefits and dangers. Let's assess the benefits and hazards of a combination of procedures for uterine prolapse:

Benefits of Combination of Procedures for Uterine Prolapse

1. <u>Holistic Treatment:</u> The combination of techniques gives for a holistic and complete approach to addressing multiple prolapse issues concurrently. This treatment can be particularly useful for women who have several pelvic organ prolapses, as it offers the chance to repair all these anomalies in a single surgical session, reducing the need for additional surgeries in the future.

2. <u>Targeted Correction:</u> By addressing distinct prolapses, the surgeon can adapt the surgeries to the unique patient's exact needs, offering targeted correction for each damaged compartment. This can result in more effective and longer-lasting outcomes.

3. <u>Minimally Invasive Techniques:</u> Depending on the severity of the prolapses and the surgeon's expertise, minimally invasive techniques such as laparoscopic or robotic-assisted surgery may be used,

leading to shorter hospital stays, less postoperative pain, and faster recovery compared to traditional open surgery.

4. <u>Potential for Preserving Uterus:</u> In instances when the patient prefers to preserve the uterus, the surgeon can often undertake surgeries to treat prolapse difficulties while retaining the uterus. This is particularly essential for women who have reproductive issues or who prefer to avoid the physiological changes associated with hysterectomy.

5. <u>Improvement of Pelvic Symptoms:</u> A successful combination of surgeries can lead to the alleviation of symptoms associated with uterine prolapse, cystocele, rectocele, and other pelvic organ prolapses. Patients commonly report alleviation from pelvic pressure, discomfort, urinary issues, and difficulties with bowel motions.

6. <u>Potential for Concurrent disorders:</u> If the patient has additional medical diseases that can be treated by surgery, such as incontinence or fibroids, these difficulties can be tackled simultaneously with prolapse correction, eliminating the need for separate surgeries.

<u>Risks and Considerations of Combination of Procedures for Uterine Prolapse</u>

1. <u>Surgical Risks:</u> As with any surgical operation, a combination of operations includes inherent surgical risks, including infection, haemorrhage, unpleasant responses to anaesthesia or medications, injury to nearby structures, and the chance of postoperative difficulties.

2. <u>Complexity:</u> Combining several operations could boost the complexity of the surgery, which may extend the surgical duration and perhaps increase the danger of certain issues. The surgeon's skill and

expertise are crucial in addressing these problems.

3. <u>Recovery Period:</u> The recovery period following a combination of therapies can be longer and more demanding compared to separate operations. The patient may have pain, limited physical activity, and limits on lifting heavy objects. The recuperation length should be thoroughly discussed with the surgeon.

4. <u>Postoperative Monitoring:</u> Patients recciving a combination of procedures should have regular follow-up visits with the surgeon to monitor the healing process, assess the success of the surgeries, and treat any complications.

5. <u>Alternative Treatments:</u> In certain instances, additional non-surgical treatments, such pelvic floor exercises, pessaries, or topical oestrogen therapy, may

be useful in managing uterine prolapse without the need for surgical intervention.

The decision to proceed with a combination of therapies should be based on a complete review of the particular circumstances, assessing the benefits against the potential hazards, and taking into account the woman's overall health, surgery history, and personal preferences.

6. <u>Hormonal Considerations: If</u> the patient undergoes a hysterectomy as part of the combination of procedures (for example, if the uterus is severely compromised or if the patient desires a hysterectomy), there may be hormonal considerations if the ovaries are removed (bilateral salpingo-oophorectomy), leading to menopause and its associated symptoms.

It's vital for women considering a combination of surgeries for uterine prolapse to have a full discussion with their healthcare provider, particularly with a gynaecologist or urogynecologist.

This consultation should thoroughly explore the benefits, hazards, and alternatives based on their individual medical history, overall health, family planning goals, and personal preferences. A personalised strategy that takes into consideration the unique conditions is crucial to making an informed selection regarding the most suitable treatment option.

SACROSPINOUS LIGAMENT SUSPENSION

In this operation, the surgeon joins the cervix or vaginal vault to the sacrospinous ligament, a strong ligament in the pelvis. This helps lift and support the uterus or vaginal vault, repairing prolapse.

Sacrospinous ligament suspension, also known as sacrospinous colpopexy, is a surgical therapy used to treat uterine prolapse and various kinds of pelvic organ prolapse (POP).

This procedure seeks to provide mechanical support to the prolapsed structures, often the vagina and uterus, by attaching them to a stable ligament within the pelvis. Sacrospinous ligament suspension is one of the several surgical treatments available to address uterine prolapse and has distinct benefits and considerations that are vital to understanding. Let's go into the details of sacrospinous ligament suspension:

Benefits of Sacrospinous Ligament Suspension for Uterine Prolapse

1. <u>Effective Support</u>: Sacrospinous ligament suspension affords effective mechanical support to the prolapsed vaginal and uterine tissues, helping to restore their natural position inside the pelvis.

2. <u>Relief from Symptoms:</u> Successful surgery can alleviate the symptoms associated with uterine prolapse, such as pelvic pressure, vaginal bulging, discomfort, urinary issues, and difficulties with bowel movements.

3. <u>Minimally intrusive:</u> The vaginal method to sacrospinous ligament suspension is less intrusive than typical abdominal operations, which often leads to shorter hospital stays, faster recovery, and lower postoperative pain.

4. <u>Preservation of Uterus:</u> Sacrospinous ligament suspension allows women who choose to preserve their uterus to avoid a hysterectomy, as the procedure focuses on offering support rather than removing the uterus.

5. <u>Potential for Combined Procedures:</u> If the patient has other concurrent prolapse disorders (e.g., cystocele, rectocele), these issues can often be addressed during the

same surgical session, giving full therapy for multiple prolapses.

Risks and Considerations of Sacrospinous Ligament Suspension

1. <u>Surgical Risks:</u> As with any surgical treatment, sacrospinous ligament suspension contains inherent surgical risks, including infection, haemorrhage, adverse reactions to anaesthesia or medicines, injury to neighbouring structures, and the chance of postoperative difficulties.

2. <u>Recurrence:</u> While sacrospinous ligament suspension helps give short-term comfort, there is a slight probability of recurrence of prolapse over time. Regular follow-up consultations with the surgeon are essential to examine the long-term consequences of the procedure.

3. <u>Recovery phase:</u> The recovery phase following sacrospinous ligament suspension could take several weeks, during which the

patient may have pain, limited physical activity, and limits on carrying heavy objects. The recuperation length should be thoroughly discussed with the surgeon.

4. <u>Alternative Treatments:</u> In certain instances, additional non-surgical treatments, such pelvic floor exercises, pessaries, or topical oestrogen therapy, may be useful in managing uterine prolapse without the need for surgical intervention.

The option to proceed with sacrospinous ligament suspension should be based on a complete examination of the particular circumstances, assessing the benefits against the potential hazards, and taking into account the woman's overall health, surgical history, and personal preferences.

5. <u>Vaginal Mesh:</u> In some cases, a surgeon may choose to deploy vaginal mesh or other synthetic materials for extra support during sacrospinous ligament suspension.

The use of vaginal mesh has been connected with unique dangers, including mesh erosion and difficulties. The decision to adopt mesh should be discussed with the surgeon, and patients should be thoroughly informed of the potential dangers and advantages.

It's vital for women considering sacrospinous ligament suspension for uterine prolapse to have a complete chat with their healthcare practitioner, ideally with a gynaecologist or urogynecologist.

This consultation should thoroughly explore the benefits, hazards, and alternatives based on their individual medical history, overall health, family planning goals, and personal preferences. A personalised strategy that takes into consideration the unique conditions is crucial to making an informed selection regarding the most suitable treatment option.

VAGINAL OBLITERATION OR COLPECTOMY

In cases when the patient is not interested in keeping vaginal function or if alternative therapies are not possible, a vaginal obliteration or colectomy may be performed. This treatment entails sealing or removing the vaginal canal, which can reduce prolapse symptoms.

Vaginal obliteration, also known as colectomy, is a surgical therapy that involves the removal or closure of the vaginal canal.

This technique is often performed for several medical objectives, including vaginal agenesis (absence or underdevelopment of the vagina), treatment of chronic vaginal infections or fistulas, or as a component of gender-affirming surgery.

Vaginal obliteration can be a vital and life-changing treatment, and it's crucial to appreciate its benefits, hazards, and precautions. Let's explore vaginal obliteration or colectomy in detail:

Benefits of Vaginal Obliteration or Colpectomy

1. <u>Functional Improvement:</u> Vaginal obliteration can address the underlying medical condition, such as vaginal agenesis, and provide a more functional pelvic architecture, allowing for improved urine and stool function in some instances.

2. <u>Resolution of Recurrent Infections:</u> For women with chronic vaginal infections, colectomy can eliminate the vaginal environment where these infections occur, leading to relief from symptoms and improved overall health.

3. <u>Treatment of Fistulas:</u> Vaginal obliteration can be a beneficial treatment for

vaginal fistulas, helping to seal the irregular pores and avoid further issues.

4. <u>Gender Affirmation:</u> For transgender individuals having MTF gender-affirming procedures, colectomy is a critical step in establishing external genitalia that agree with their gender identification, adding to overall psychological well-being.

Risks and Considerations of Vaginal Obliteration or Colpectomy

1. <u>Irreversible:</u> Vaginal obliteration is an irreversible procedure. Once the vaginal canal is closed, it cannot be reopened. Therefore, careful evaluation and counselling are essential, especially for women who may choose to have vaginal intercourse in the future or for whom keeping the possibility of pregnancy is crucial.

2. <u>Impair on Sexual Function:</u> Vaginal obliteration can impair sexual function and may affect sexual experiences. Patients must express their sexual health aspirations and concerns with their healthcare practitioner.

3. <u>Psychological Impact:</u> The decision to undergo vaginal obliteration, particularly as part of gender-affirming surgeries, has serious psychological repercussions. Individuals need to undergo comprehensive therapy and guidance from mental health experts skilled in gender identity and surgical concerns.

4. <u>Recovery and Healing:</u> As with any surgical treatment, recovery following vaginal obliteration entails a healing phase, during which patients may suffer discomfort, vaginal bleeding, or other postoperative symptoms.

5. <u>Other Treatments:</u> In some instances, other treatments or therapies, such as

dilator therapy or hormonal interventions, may be suitable for treating the medical condition without the need for surgical intervention. These choices should be addressed with the healthcare provider.

6. <u>Potential challenges:</u> While vaginal obliteration is normally a safe surgery, it has intrinsic surgical risks, such as infection, bleeding, anaesthesia difficulties, and poor responses to medicines.

Vaginal obliteration or colectomy is a surgical method with unique indications, benefits, and considerations. It's vital for people considering this surgery to have a complete chat with their healthcare practitioner, ideally with a gynaecologist or a surgeon knowledgeable in gender-affirming surgeries if available.

The selection should be based on a complete examination of the particular medical condition, individual goals, general health, psychological issues, and personal preferences. A personalised strategy that takes into account the individual conditions and potential long-term impact is crucial to making an informed selection regarding the most suitable treatment method.

ROBOTIC-ASSISTED SURGERY

Robotic-assisted surgery is a minimally invasive treatment that offers increased precision and visualisation for the physician. This method may be applied for hysterectomy, sacral colpopexy, or other surgical procedures to treat uterine prolapse.

Robotic-assisted surgery has grown as a technologically improved alternative for various gynaecological operations, including the treatment of uterine prolapse.

This novel surgical treatment, also known as a robot-assisted laparoscopic surgery, utilises advanced robotic equipment to assist doctors in conducting challenging surgeries with increased precision and flexibility. Robotic-assisted surgery for uterine prolapse offers numerous benefits, along with particular precautions and potential risks. Let's investigate this topic in detail:

<u>Benefits of Robotic-Assisted Surgery for Uterine Prolapse</u>

1. <u>Accurate Tissue Manipulation:</u> The robotic system's articulated instruments allow the surgeon to manipulate tissue with higher accuracy, enabling more accurate repairs of weakened pelvic tissues during uterine prolapse surgery.

2. <u>High-Definition Visualisation:</u> The 3D visualisation given by the robotic system enhances the surgeon's capacity to notice minute details, which is crucial in identifying and correcting prolapse-related problems.

3. <u>Lower Blood Loss:</u> The minimally invasive nature of robotic-assisted surgery typically leads to lower blood loss throughout the procedure, contributing to improved patient outcomes.

4. <u>Faster Recovery:</u> Patients getting robotic-assisted surgery for uterine prolapse often report a speedier recovery, allowing them to return to their regular activities sooner.

5. <u>Lower Risk of Infection:</u> Smaller incisions and reduced tissue stress may result in a lower risk of postoperative infections compared to open operations.

6. <u>Preservation of Uterus:</u> For women who choose to save their uterus, robotic-assisted surgery can present a less intrusive approach to address uterine prolapse while retaining the uterus.

<u>Considerations and Potential Risks</u>

1. <u>Surgeon expertise:</u> The effectiveness of robotic-assisted surgery depends on the surgeon's expertise and ability with the robotic system. Patients should select surgeons who are trained and skilled in robotic-assisted procedures.

2. <u>Cost:</u> Robotic-assisted surgery may be more expensive than standard laparoscopic or open surgeries due to the particular equipment and technology needed. Patients should review the cost and potential insurance coverage with their healthcare professional.

3. <u>Operative Time:</u> Robotic-assisted operations may take longer than traditional laparoscopic procedures, which can affect anaesthesia duration and overall operating room time.

4.   <u>Postoperative   Care:</u>   While robotic-assisted surgery is minimally invasive, patients still need to follow postoperative care procedures to ensure a smooth recovery. It's vital to adhere to the surgeon's directions for physical exercise, wound care, and follow-up consultations.

5. <u>Technology Availability:</u> Not all healthcare facilities have access to robotic-assisted surgical technologies. Patients interested in this method may inquire about the availability of the technology at their designated healthcare practitioner.

6. <u>Potential challenges:</u> As with any surgical operation, robotic-assisted surgery involves inherent surgical hazards, including infection, bleeding, anaesthesia difficulties, and poor reactions to medicines.

7. <u>Alternative Treatments:</u> In certain instances, other treatment approaches,

including pelvic floor exercises, pessaries, or topical oestrogen therapy, may be useful in reducing uterine prolapse without the need for invasive surgery.

The decision to proceed with robotic-assisted surgery should be based on a complete analysis of the unique circumstance, contrasting the benefits against the potential hazards, and taking into account the woman's overall health, surgical history, and personal preferences.

Robotic-assisted surgery offers several advantages for the treatment of uterine prolapse, including improved precision, the least intrusive procedure, and quicker recovery.

Patients contemplating this procedure should visit with a qualified surgeon versed in robotic-assisted surgeries and have a full chat about the potential advantages, risks, and alternatives. A personalised approach, taking into account the individual's medical history, overall health, and preferences, is crucial to making an informed decision regarding the best-suited treatment option for uterine prolapse.

PREOPERATIVE EVALUATION

Before having any surgical operation, a complete preoperative evaluation is conducted to check the patient's overall health, including factors such as heart and lung function. This assessment helps identify the appropriate surgical method and reduce potential hazards.

Benefits of Preoperative Evaluation for Uterine Prolapse

1. <u>Customised Surgical Approach:</u> A thorough preoperative evaluation allows the healthcare team to adjust the surgical approach to the particular needs of the patient. The evaluation helps define the most appropriate surgical technique, taking into account the severity of prolapse, the

patient's overall health, and any concurrent pelvic illnesses.

2. <u>Enhanced Safety:</u> Identifying any underlying medical concerns or risk factors before surgery enables the healthcare team to take appropriate safeguards, limit surgical risks, and optimise the patient's safety during the procedure and throughout the recovery period.

3. <u>Optimal Surgical Outcomes:</u> By addressing medical issues and enhancing the patient's health before surgery, the preoperative evaluation can lead to superior surgical outcomes. This includes decreasing the chance of problems, providing a speedier recovery, and enhancing the overall success of the uterine prolapse operation.

4. <u>Informed Decision-Making:</u> Through the preoperative assessment, the healthcare professional educates the patient about the surgical process, explains potential risks and

advantages, and delivers the necessary knowledge for the patient to make an informed decision about the treatment. This informed consent strategy is crucial for patient autonomy and enjoyment.

5. <u>Identification of Concurrent Issues:</u> A complete evaluation may identify concurrent pelvic floor abnormalities, such as bladder or rectal prolapse, that may demand concurrent procedures. Addressing several problems during a single surgery can be more efficient for the patient, minimising the need for repeated surgeries in the future.

6. <u>Anaesthetic Management:</u> The anaesthetic evaluation during the preoperative assessment ensures that the patient is well-prepared for anaesthesia, minimising the risk of complications associated with anaesthesia administration. Anaesthesia doctors can personalise the anaesthesia approach to the patient's medical history and preferences.

<u>Risks and Considerations of Preoperative Evaluation for Uterine Prolapse</u>

1. <u>Time and Resources:</u> A thorough preoperative evaluation may take additional time and resources, including consultations, laboratory testing, imaging studies, and anaesthetic evaluations. However, these investments are important for maintaining patient safety and surgical success.

2. <u>Worry and Uncertainty:</u> The preoperative evaluation process can occasionally add to greater worry for the patient, especially if they are inexperienced with the surgical process or if concerns surface during the evaluation. Effective communication and patient education can help ease these worries.

3. <u>Potential for Delay:</u> In some circumstances, the preoperative evaluation may identify medical concerns that need to

be addressed before the surgery can commence. This may result in a temporary delay in the surgical schedule to provide time for optimization of the patient's health.

4. <u>False Positives:</u> In rare cases, the preoperative screening may identify possible issues that, upon deeper scrutiny, turn out to be false positives or not clinically meaningful. This problem can lead to needless further testing or consultations.

5. <u>Patient Anxiety:</u> While the preoperative evaluation is designed to deliver detailed information and raise patient awareness, it may also add to anxiety about the surgery or concerns about the revealed medical issues. Healthcare providers should address these difficulties and give the necessary support.

6. <u>Unforeseen issues:</u> Despite comprehensive preoperative assessment, there is still the potential of unforeseen difficulties during the procedure. However,

a well-conducted examination minimise these risks by identifying and resolving recognized causes.

The benefits of a complete preoperative assessment for uterine prolapse far transcend the potential dangers and considerations. A well-planned and thorough examination ensures that the patient is completely prepared for surgery, minimises surgical risks, and promotes optimal surgical outcomes.

Open communication between the patient, surgeon, and healthcare team is crucial to address any concerns and ensure that the patient has a full grasp of the preoperative evaluation process and its usefulness. Ultimately, the preoperative assessment plays a significant role in the complete care of uterine prolapse, contributing to a safe and productive surgical experience.

Tailored Treatment Plans: Each patient's scenario is unique, and a tailored treatment plan is crucial for optimal outcomes. A healthcare provider will assess the patient's age, overall health, desire for future pregnancies, severity of prolapse, and personal preferences while offering the most suitable intervention.

Benefits of Individualised Treatment Plans for Uterine Prolapse

1.   Tailored Approach: Individualised treatment approaches take into account the unique characteristics of each patient, such as the severity of uterine prolapse, overall health, medical history, pelvic anatomy, age, lifestyle, and personal preferences. This personalised approach guarantees that the treatment matches the specific expectations of the client.

2.   Optimal Treatment Selection: By examining the unique patient's circumstances, the healthcare provider can

choose the most appropriate treatment option for uterine prolapse. This may involve non-surgical treatments, minimally invasive procedures, or more substantial surgeries, depending on what best suits the patient's goals and medical condition.

3. <u>Patient Satisfaction:</u> When patients are actively involved in the decision-making process and given treatment alternatives adapted to their preferences and lifestyle, they are more likely to be satisfied with the chosen approach and the overall outcomes of the therapy.

4. <u>Improved Quality of Life:</u> A personalised treatment strategy takes into account not only the physical components of uterine prolapse but also its impact on the patient's quality of life. By addressing the individual symptoms and concerns that matter most to the patient, the treatment plan seeks to promote overall well-being.

5. <u>Maximising Non-Surgical Options:</u> In cases where the severity of uterine prolapse allows for non-surgical management, an individualised treatment plan can explore and maximise the effectiveness of conservative measures, such as pelvic floor exercises, pessaries, and hormone therapy, before considering more invasive interventions.

6. <u>Consideration of Future Goals:</u> The patient's future goals, such as fertility ambitions or concerns about sexual function, might be carefully considered in the individualised treatment plan. For women who wish to retain fertility or maintain sexual function, choices that align with these aspirations can be considered.

<u>Risks and Considerations of Individualised Treatment Plans for Uterine Prolapse</u>

1. <u>Complex Decision-Making:</u> Individualised treatment regimens need thorough

evaluation and consideration of multiple parameters. This complexity can frequently make the decision-making process more confusing for the patient and the healthcare provider.

2. <u>Potential for Delay:</u> In cases when there are multiple treatment possibilities to consider, obtaining a final decision may take some time. This delay could alter the timing of treatment, particularly if surgical intervention is necessary.

3. <u>Variability in Outcomes:</u> The success of a personalised treatment plan depends on various elements, including the patient's dedication to the plan, the chosen treatment's effectiveness, and the natural course of uterine prolapse. Outcomes may vary, and certain medicines may require continual monitoring.

4. <u>Patient Education:</u> Individualised treatment regimens entail rigorous patient

education to ensure that the patient knows the therapy alternatives, potential risks, advantages, and expected outcomes. Adequate patient education is crucial for shared decision-making.

5. <u>Risk of Treatment Overload:</u> In rare instances, the amount of available treatment alternatives may contribute to information overload for the patient. It's vital to give the options in a straightforward and manageable format, allowing the patient to make educated selections without feeling overwhelmed.

6. <u>Changing Circumstances:</u> Patients' circumstances and preferences may fluctuate over time, leading to the need for adjustments to the treatment plan. The healthcare practitioner should stay open to continuing communication and periodic reevaluation.

The benefits of personalised treatment strategies for uterine prolapse, which include customising the approach to the patient's particular needs and maximising treatment selection, are crucial.

Although there are considerations and potential hazards, the customised method strives to deliver the best possible outcomes, raise patient satisfaction, and improve the overall quality of life.

Open communication between the patient and healthcare provider, collaborative decision-making, and constant review are key features of the success of personalised treatment solutions for uterine prolapse.

POSTOPERATIVE CARE AND FOLLOW-UP

After surgical intervention, adequate postoperative care and follow-up are required. Patients should comply with recovery guidelines supplied by their healthcare practitioner, which may include restrictions on physical activity, sufficient wound care, and planned follow-up consultations to monitor healing and treat any concerns.

Alternative Therapies

Some folks investigate alternative therapies, such as physical therapy, acupuncture, or herbal cures. While these therapies may offer some comfort or augment regular treatments, it's crucial to discuss their use with a healthcare specialist to verify they are safe and effective in the specific context of uterine prolapse.

It's crucial to stress that the option of medical or surgical intervention depends on the individual's personal circumstances, choices, and medical concerns.

A thorough discussion with a healthcare practitioner, including a clear grasp of the benefits, dangers, and expected outcomes, is crucial in making informed decisions regarding the best appropriate treatment option for uterine prolapse.